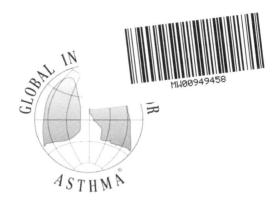

GLOBAL INITIATIVE FOR ASTHMA

ASTHMA MANAGEMENT AND PREVENTION
for adults and children older than 5 years

A POCKET GUIDE FOR HEALTH PROFESSIONALS

Updated 2019

GINA Science Committee
Chair: Helen Reddel, MBBS PhD

GINA Board of Directors
Chair: Louis-Philippe Boulet, MD

GINA Dissemination and Implementation Committee
Chair: Mark Levy, MBChB

GINA Assembly
The GINA Assembly includes members from 45 countries, listed on the GINA website www.ginasthma.org.

GINA Program Director
Rebecca Decker, BS, MSJ

Names of members of the GINA Committees are listed on page 36.

A MAJOR CHANGE IN THE GINA 2019 STRATEGY

The 2019 GINA strategy report represents the most important change in asthma management in 30 years.

For safety, GINA no longer recommends treatment with short-acting beta2-agonists (SABA) alone. There is strong evidence that SABA-only treatment, although providing short-term relief of asthma symptoms, does not protect patients from severe exacerbations, and that regular or frequent use of SABAs increases the risk of exacerbations.

GINA now recommends that all adults and adolescents with asthma should receive either symptom-driven or regular low dose ICS-containing controller treatment, to reduce their risk of serious exacerbations.

Details about the new treatment recommendations, and the rationale for the new recommendations, begin on page 16, with the new treatment figure on page 19. Information about ICS doses is found on page 20.

Why has GINA changed its recommendations for mild asthma?

These new recommendations represent the culmination of a 12-year campaign by GINA to obtain evidence for strategies to improve the treatment of mild asthma. Our aims were:

- to reduce the risk of serious asthma-related exacerbations and death, including in patients with so-called mild asthma,
- to provide consistent messaging about the aims of asthma treatment, including prevention of exacerbations, across the whole spectrum of asthma severity
- to avoid establishing a pattern of patient reliance on SABA early in the course of the disease.

LIST OF ABBREVIATIONS

BDP	Beclometasone dipropionate
COPD	Chronic obstructive pulmonary disease
CXR	Chest X-ray
DPI	Dry powder inhaler
FeNO	Fraction of exhaled nitric oxide
FEV_1	Forced expiratory volume in 1 second
FVC	Forced vital capacity
GERD	Gastroesophageal reflux disease
HDM	House dust mite
ICS	Inhaled corticosteroids
Ig	Immunoglobulin
IL	Interleukin
IV	Intravenous
LABA	Long-acting beta$_2$-agonist
LAMA	Long-acting muscarinic antagonist
LTRA	Leukotriene receptor antagonist
n.a.	Not applicable
NSAID	Non-steroidal anti-inflammatory drug
O_2	Oxygen
OCS	Oral corticosteroids
PEF	Peak expiratory flow
pMDI	Pressurized metered dose inhaler
SABA	Short-acting beta$_2$-agonist
SC	Subcutaneous
SLIT	Sublingual immunotherapy

TABLE OF CONTENTS

TABLE OF FIGURES

ABOUT GINA

Asthma affects an estimated 300 million individuals worldwide. It is a serious global health problem affecting all age groups, with increasing prevalence in many developing countries, rising treatment costs, and a rising burden for patients and the community. Asthma still imposes an unacceptable burden on health care systems, and on society through loss of productivity in the workplace and, especially for pediatric asthma, disruption to the family, and it still contributes to many deaths worldwide, including among young people.

Health care providers managing asthma face different issues globally, depending on the local context, the health system, and access to resources.

The **Global Initiative for Asthma (GINA)** was established to increase awareness about asthma among health professionals, public health authorities and the community, and to improve prevention and management through a coordinated worldwide effort. GINA prepares scientific reports on asthma, encourages dissemination and implementation of the recommendations, and promotes international collaboration on asthma research.

The **Global Strategy for Asthma Management and Prevention** provides a comprehensive and integrated approach to asthma management that can be adapted for local conditions and for individual patients. It focuses not only on the existing strong evidence base, but also on clarity of language and on providing tools for feasible implementation in clinical practice. The report is updated each year. **The 2019 GINA report includes important new recommendations for treatment of mild asthma (page 16) and severe asthma (page 24).**

The GINA 2019 report and other GINA publications listed on page 36 can be obtained from www.ginasthma.org.

The reader acknowledges that this **Pocket Guide** is a brief summary of the GINA 2019 report, for primary health care providers. It does NOT contain all of the information required for managing asthma, for example, about safety of treatments, and it should be used in conjunction with the full GINA 2019 report and with the health professional's own clinical judgment. GINA cannot be held liable or responsible for inappropriate healthcare associated with the use of this document, including any use which is not in accordance with applicable local or national regulations or guidelines.

WHAT IS KNOWN ABOUT ASTHMA?

Asthma is a common and potentially serious chronic disease that imposes a substantial burden on patients, their families and the community. It causes respiratory symptoms, limitation of activity, and flare-ups (attacks) that sometimes require urgent health care and may be fatal.

Fortunately...asthma can be effectively treated, and most patients can achieve good control of their asthma. When asthma is under good control, patients can:
- ✓ Avoid troublesome symptoms during day and night
- ✓ Need little or no reliever medication
- ✓ Have productive, physically active lives
- ✓ Have normal or near normal lung function
- ✓ Avoid serious asthma flare-ups (exacerbations, or attacks)

What is asthma? Asthma causes symptoms such as wheezing, shortness of breath, chest tightness and cough that vary over time in their occurrence, frequency and intensity. These symptoms are associated with variable expiratory airflow, i.e. difficulty breathing air out of the lungs due to bronchoconstriction (airway narrowing), airway wall thickening, and increased mucus. Some variation in airflow can also occur in people without asthma, but it is greater in asthma before treatment is started. There are different types of asthma, with different underlying disease processes.

Factors that may trigger or worsen asthma symptoms include viral infections, allergens at home or work (e.g. house dust mite, pollens, cockroach), tobacco smoke, exercise and stress. These responses are more likely when asthma is uncontrolled. Some drugs can induce or trigger asthma, e.g. beta-blockers, and (in some patients), aspirin or other NSAIDs.

Asthma flare-ups (also called exacerbations or attacks) can be fatal. They are more common and more severe when asthma is uncontrolled, or in some high-risk patients. However, flare-ups may occur even in people taking asthma treatment, so all patients should have an asthma action plan.

Treatment with inhaled corticosteroid (ICS)-containing medications markedly reduces the frequency and severity of asthma symptoms and markedly reduces the risk of flare-ups or dying of asthma.

Asthma treatment should be customized to the individual patient, taking into account their level of symptom control, their risk factors for exacerbations, phenotypic characteristics, and preferences, as well as the effectiveness of available medications, their safety, and their cost to the payer or patient.

Asthma is a common condition, affecting all levels of society. Olympic athletes, famous leaders and celebrities, and ordinary people live **successful and active lives with asthma**.

MAKING THE DIAGNOSIS OF ASTHMA

Asthma is a disease with many variations (heterogeneous), usually characterized by chronic airway inflammation. Asthma has two key defining features:

- a history of respiratory symptoms such as wheeze, shortness of breath, chest tightness and cough that vary over time and in intensity, AND
- variable expiratory airflow limitation.

A flow-chart for making the diagnosis in clinical practice is shown in Box 1, with the specific criteria for diagnosing asthma in Box 2.

Box 1. Diagnostic flow-chart for asthma in clinical practice

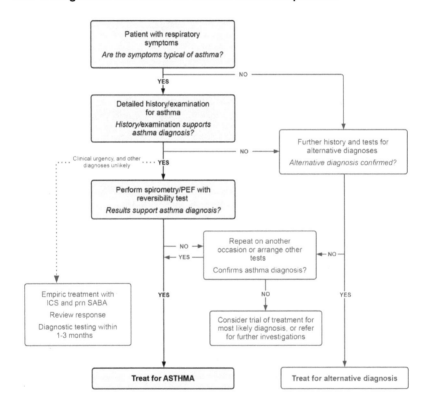

The **diagnosis of asthma** should be confirmed and, for future reference, the evidence documented in the patient's notes. This should preferably be done before starting controller treatment. Confirming the diagnosis of asthma is more difficult after treatment has been started (see p11).

CRITERIA FOR MAKING THE DIAGNOSIS OF ASTHMA

Box 2. Features used in making the diagnosis of asthma

1. A history of variable respiratory symptoms

Typical symptoms are wheeze, shortness of breath, chest tightness, cough
- People with asthma generally have more than one of these symptoms
- The symptoms occur variably over time and vary in intensity
- The symptoms often occur or are worse at night or on waking
- Symptoms are often triggered by exercise, laughter, allergens or cold air
- Symptoms often occur with or worsen with viral infections

2. Evidence of variable expiratory airflow limitation

- At least once during the diagnostic process, e.g. when FEV_1 is low, document that the FEV_1/FVC ratio is below the lower limit of normal[†]. The FEV_1/FVC ratio is normally more than 0.75–0.80 in adults, and more than 0.85 in children.

- Document that variation in lung function is greater than in healthy people. For example, excess variability is recorded if:
  - FEV_1 increases by >200mL and >12% of the baseline value (or in children, increases by >12% of the predicted value) after inhaling a bronchodilator. This is called 'bronchodilator reversibility'.
  - Average daily diurnal PEF variability* is >10% (in children, >13%)
  - FEV_1 increases by more than 12% and 200mL from baseline (in children, by >12% of the predicted value) after 4 weeks of anti-inflammatory treatment (outside respiratory infections)

- The greater the variation, or the more times excess variation is seen, the more confident you can be of the diagnosis of asthma.

- Testing may need to be repeated during symptoms, in the early morning, or after withholding bronchodilator medications.

- Bronchodilator reversibility may be absent during severe exacerbations or viral infections. If bronchodilator reversibility is not present when it is first tested, the next step depends on the clinical urgency and the availability of other tests.

- For other tests to assist in diagnosis, including bronchial challenge tests, see Chapter 1 of the GINA 2019 report.

*Calculated from twice daily readings (best of 3 each time), as (the day's highest PEF minus the day's lowest PEF) divided by the mean of the day's highest and lowest PEF, and averaged over 1-2 weeks. If using PEF at home or in the office, use the same PEF meter each time. † Using Global Lung Initiative multi-ethnic reference equations.

Physical examination in people with asthma is often normal, but the most frequent finding is wheezing on auscultation, especially on forced expiration.

HOW TO CONFIRM THE DIAGNOSIS IN PATIENTS TAKING CONTROLLER TREATMENT

For many patients (25–35%) with a diagnosis of asthma in primary care, the diagnosis cannot be confirmed. If the basis of the diagnosis has not already been documented, confirmation with objective testing should be sought.

If standard criteria for asthma (Box 2, p.9) are not met, consider other investigations. For example, if lung function is normal, repeat reversibility testing when the patient is symptomatic, or after withholding bronchodilator medications for >12 hours (24 hours if ultra-long-acting). If the patient has frequent symptoms, consider a trial of step-up in controller treatment and repeat lung function testing after 3 months. If the patient has few symptoms, consider stepping down controller treatment; ensure the patient has a written asthma action plan, monitor them carefully, and repeat lung function testing.

DIAGNOSING ASTHMA IN OTHER CONTEXTS

Occupational asthma and work-aggravated asthma

Every patient with adult-onset asthma should be asked about occupational exposures, and whether their asthma is better when they are away from work. It is important to confirm the diagnosis objectively (which often needs specialist referral) and to eliminate exposure as quickly as possible.

Pregnant women

Ask all pregnant women and those planning pregnancy about asthma, and advise them about the importance of taking asthma controller treatment for the health of both mother and baby.

The elderly

Asthma may be under-diagnosed in the elderly, due to poor perception, an assumption that dyspnea is normal in old age, lack of fitness, or reduced activity. Asthma may also be over-diagnosed in the elderly through confusion with shortness of breath due to left ventricular failure or ischemic heart disease. If there is a history of smoking or biomass fuel exposure, COPD or asthma-COPD overlap should be considered (see below).

Smokers and ex-smokers

Asthma and COPD may co-exist or overlap (asthma-COPD overlap), particularly in smokers and the elderly. The history and pattern of symptoms and past records can help to distinguish asthma with persistent airflow limitation from COPD. Uncertainty in diagnosis should prompt early referral, because asthma-COPD overlap has worse outcomes than asthma or COPD alone. Asthma-COPD overlap is not a single disease, but is likely caused by several different mechanisms. There is little randomized controlled trial evidence about how to treat these patients, as they are often excluded from clinical trials. However, given the risks associated with treating with bronchodilators alone in patients with asthma, patients with COPD should be treated with at least low dose ICS (see p.20) if there is any history of asthma or diagnosis of asthma.

Patients with cough as the only respiratory symptom

This may be due to chronic upper airway cough syndrome ('post-nasal drip'), chronic sinusitis, gastroesophageal reflux (GERD), inducible laryngeal obstruction (often called vocal cord dysfunction), eosinophilic bronchitis, or cough variant asthma. Cough variant asthma is characterized by cough and airway hyperresponsiveness, and documenting variability in lung function is essential to make this diagnosis. However, lack of variability at the time of testing does not exclude asthma. For other diagnostic tests, see Box 2, and Chapter 1 of the GINA 2019 report, or refer the patient for specialist opinion.

ASSESSING A PATIENT WITH ASTHMA

Take every opportunity to assess patients with asthma, particularly when they are symptomatic or after a recent exacerbation, but also when they ask for a prescription refill. In addition, schedule a routine review at least once a year.

Box 3. How to assess a patient with asthma

1. Asthma control – assess both symptom control and risk factors
<ul><li>Assess symptom control over the last 4 weeks (Box 4, p12)</li><li>Identify any modifiable risk factors for poor outcomes (Box 4)</li><li>Measure lung function before starting treatment, 3–6 months later, and then periodically, e.g. at least yearly in most patients</li></ul>
2. Are there any comorbidities?
<ul><li>These include rhinitis, chronic rhinosinusitis, gastroesophageal reflux (GERD), obesity, obstructive sleep apnea, depression and anxiety.</li><li>Comorbidities should be identified as they may contribute to respiratory symptoms, flare-ups and poor quality of life. Their treatment may complicate asthma management.</li></ul>
3. Treatment issues
<ul><li>Record the patient's treatment (Box 7, p.19), and ask about side-effects</li><li>Watch the patient using their inhaler, to check their technique (p.26)</li><li>Have an open empathic discussion about adherence (p.26)</li><li>Check that the patient has a written asthma action plan (p.29)</li><li>Ask the patient about their attitudes and goals for their asthma</li></ul>

HOW TO ASSESS ASTHMA CONTROL

Asthma control means the extent to which the effects of asthma can be seen in the patient, or have been reduced or removed by treatment. Asthma control has two domains: symptom control and risk factors for future poor outcomes, particularly flare-ups (exacerbations). Questionnaires like Asthma Control Test and Asthma Control Questionnaire assess only symptom control.

Poor symptom control is a burden to patients and a risk factor for flare-ups. **Risk factors** are factors that increase the patient's future risk of having exacerbations (flare-ups), loss of lung function, or medication side-effects.

Box 4. Assessment of symptom control and future risk

A. Level of asthma symptom control

In the past 4 weeks, has the patient had:		Well controlled	Partly controlled	Uncontrolled
Daytime symptoms more than twice/week?	Yes☐ No☐			
Any night waking due to asthma?	Yes☐ No☐	None	1–2	3–4
Reliever needed more than twice/week?	Yes☐ No☐	of these	of these	of these
Any activity limitation due to asthma?	Yes☐ No☐			

B. Risk factors for poor asthma outcomes

Assess risk factors at diagnosis and periodically, at least every 1-2 years, particularly for patients experiencing exacerbations.

Measure FEV_1 at start of treatment, after 3–6 months of controller treatment to record personal best lung function, then periodically for ongoing risk assessment.

Having uncontrolled asthma symptoms is an important risk factor for exacerbations

Additional potentially modifiable risk factors for exacerbations, even in patients with few asthma symptoms, include:

Having any of these risk factors increases the patient's risk of exacerbations *even if they have few asthma symptoms.*

- *Medications*: ICS not prescribed; poor adherence; incorrect inhaler technique; high SABA use (with increased mortality if >1x200-dose canister/month)
- *Comorbidities*: obesity; chronic rhinosinusitis; gastro-esophageal reflux disease; confirmed food allergy; anxiety; depression; pregnancy
- *Exposures*: smoking; allergen exposure if sensitized; air pollution
- *Setting*: major socioeconomic problems
- *Lung function*: low FEV_1, especially if <60% predicted; higher reversibility
- *Other tests*: sputum/blood eosinophilia; elevated FENO in allergic adults on ICS

Other major independent risk factors for flare-ups (exacerbations) include:
- Ever being intubated or in intensive care for asthma
- Having 1 or more severe exacerbations in the last 12 months.

Risk factors for developing fixed airflow limitation include preterm birth, low birth weight and greater infant weight gain; lack of ICS treatment; exposure to tobacco smoke, noxious chemicals or occupational exposures; low FEV_1; chronic mucus hypersecretion; and sputum or blood eosinophilia

Risk factors for medication side-effects include:
- *Systemic*: frequent OCS; long-term, high dose and/or potent ICS; also taking P450 inhibitors
- *Local*: high-dose or potent ICS; poor inhaler technique

ICS: short-acting b_2-agonist; OCS: oral corticosteroid; SABA: short-acting b_2-agonist

What is the role of lung function in monitoring asthma?

Once asthma has been diagnosed, lung function is most useful as an indicator of future risk. It should be recorded at diagnosis, 3–6 months after starting treatment, and periodically thereafter. Most patients should have lung function measured at least every 1-2 years, more often in children and those at higher risk of flare-ups or lung function decline. Patients who have either few or many symptoms relative to their lung function need more investigation.

How is asthma severity assessed?

Currently, asthma severity is assessed retrospectively from the level of treatment (p.19) required to control symptoms and exacerbations. Mild asthma is asthma that can be controlled with Step 1 or 2 treatment. Severe asthma is asthma that requires Step 5 treatment. It may appear similar to asthma that is uncontrolled due to lack of treatment.

HOW TO INVESTIGATE UNCONTROLLED ASTHMA

Most patients can achieve good asthma control with regular controller treatment, but some patients do not, and further investigation is needed.

Box 5. How to investigate uncontrolled asthma in primary care

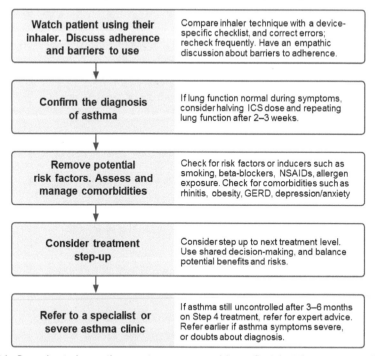

Watch patient using their inhaler. Discuss adherence and barriers to use	Compare inhaler technique with a device-specific checklist, and correct errors; recheck frequently. Have an empathic discussion about barriers to adherence.
Confirm the diagnosis of asthma	If lung function normal during symptoms, consider halving ICS dose and repeating lung function after 2–3 weeks.
Remove potential risk factors. Assess and manage comorbidities	Check for risk factors or inducers such as smoking, beta-blockers, NSAIDs, allergen exposure. Check for comorbidities such as rhinitis, obesity, GERD, depression/anxiety
Consider treatment step-up	Consider step up to next treatment level. Use shared decision-making, and balance potential benefits and risks.
Refer to a specialist or severe asthma clinic	If asthma still uncontrolled after 3–6 months on Step 4 treatment, refer for expert advice. Refer earlier if asthma symptoms severe, or doubts about diagnosis.

This flow-chart shows the most common problems first, but the steps can be carried out in a different order, depending on resources and clinical context.

MANAGEMENT OF ASTHMA

GENERAL PRINCIPLES

The long-term goals of asthma management are **risk reduction** and **symptom control**. The aim is to reduce the burden to the patient and to reduce their risk of asthma-related death, exacerbations, airway damage, and medication side-effects. The patient's own goals regarding their asthma and its treatment should also be identified.

Population-level recommendations about 'preferred' asthma treatments represent the best treatment for most patients in a population.

Patient-level treatment decisions should take into account any individual characteristics, risk factors, comorbidities or phenotype that predict the patient's likely response to treatment in terms of their symptoms and exacerbation risk, together with their personal goals, and practical issues such as inhaler technique, adherence, and affordability.

A **partnership** between the patient and their health care providers is important for effective asthma management. Training health care providers in **communication skills** may lead to increased patient satisfaction, better health outcomes, and reduced use of health care resources.

Health literacy – that is, the patient's ability to obtain, process and understand basic health information to make appropriate health decisions – should be taken into account in asthma management and education.

THE ASTHMA MANAGEMENT CYCLE TO MINIMIZE RISK AND CONTROL SYMPTOMS

Asthma management involves a continuous cycle to **assess**, **adjust treatment** and **review response** (see Box 6, p.x).

Assessment of a patient with asthma includes not only **symptom control**, but also the patient's individual **risk factors and comorbidities** that can contribute to their burden of disease and risk of poor health outcomes, or that may predict their response to treatment. The asthma-related **goals** of the patient (and of the parent(s) of children with asthma) should also be elicited.

Treatment to prevent asthma exacerbations and control symptoms includes:
- Medications: GINA now recommends that every adult and adolescent with asthma should receive ICS-containing controller medication to reduce their risk of serious exacerbations, even in patients with infrequent symptoms. Every patient with asthma should have a reliever inhaler.
- Treat modifiable risk factors and comorbidities
- Use non-pharmacological therapies and strategies as appropriate

Importantly, every patient should also be trained in **essential skills** and guided asthma self-management, including:
- Asthma information
- Inhaler skills (p26)
- Adherence (p26)
- Written asthma action plan (p29)
- Self-monitoring of symptoms and/or peak flow
- Regular medical review (p11)

The patient's **response** should be evaluated whenever treatment is changed. Assess symptom control, exacerbations, side-effects, lung function and patient (and parent, for children with asthma) satisfaction.

Box 6. The asthma management cycle to prevent exacerbations and control symptoms

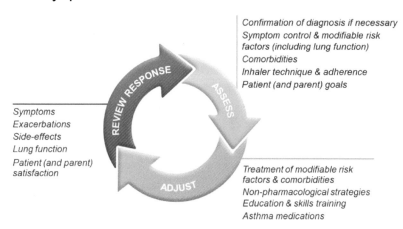

Confirmation of diagnosis if necessary
Symptom control & modifiable risk factors (including lung function)
Comorbidities
Inhaler technique & adherence
Patient (and parent) goals

Symptoms
Exacerbations
Side-effects
Lung function
Patient (and parent) satisfaction

Treatment of modifiable risk factors & comorbidities
Non-pharmacological strategies
Education & skills training
Asthma medications

A MAJOR CHANGE IN GINA 2019 RECOMMENDATIONS FOR MILD ASTHMA

From 2019, for safety, GINA no longer recommends starting with SABA-only treatment. GINA recommends that all adults and adolescents with asthma should receive ICS-containing controller treatment, to reduce their risk of serious exacerbations and to control symptoms.

Box 7 (p.19) shows the new ICS controller options. These now include:

- (for mild asthma) as-needed low dose ICS-formoterol*, or if not available, low dose ICS taken whenever SABA is taken†, or
- regular ICS or ICS-LABA every day, plus as-needed SABA, or
- maintenance and reliever treatment with ICS-formoterol, with the reliever being low-dose budesonide-formoterol or BDP-formoterol.

*Off-label; evidence only with budesonide-formoterol; †Off-label, combination or separate inhalers. For ICS dose ranges, see Box 8, p.20.

Why has GINA changed these recommendations?

The new recommendations represent the culmination of a 12-year campaign by GINA to obtain evidence for new strategies for treatment of mild asthma. Our aims were:

- to reduce the risk of asthma-related exacerbations and death, including in patients with so-called mild asthma,
- to provide consistent messaging about the aims of treatment, including prevention of exacerbations, across the spectrum of asthma severity
- to avoid establishing a pattern of patient reliance on SABA early in the course of the disease.

Additional information is provided on page 21 about the evidence and rationale for each of the new recommendations in Steps 1 and 2.

Why are there concerns about SABA-only treatment?

Many guidelines recommend that patients with mild asthma should be treated with as-needed SABA reliever alone. This dates back more than 50 years, to when asthma was thought of primarily as a disease of bronchoconstriction. However, airway inflammation is found in most patients with asthma, even in those with intermittent or infrequent symptoms.

Although SABA provides quick relief of symptoms, SABA-only treatment is associated with increased risk of exacerbations and lower lung function. Regular use increases allergic responses and airway inflammation. Over-use of SABA (e.g. ≥3 canisters dispensed in a year) is associated with an increased risk of severe exacerbations, and dispensing of ≥12 canisters in a year is associated with increased risk of asthma-related death.

STARTING ASTHMA TREATMENT

For the best outcomes, ICS-containing treatment should be initiated as soon as possible after the diagnosis of asthma is made, because:

- Patients with even mild asthma can have severe exacerbations
- Low dose ICS markedly reduces asthma hospitalizations and death
- Low dose ICS is very effective in preventing severe exacerbations, reducing symptoms, improving lung function, and preventing exercise-induced bronchoconstriction, even in patients with mild asthma
- Early treatment with low dose ICS leads to better lung function than if symptoms have been present for more than 2–4 years
- Patients not taking ICS who experience a severe exacerbation have lower long-term lung function than those who have started ICS
- In occupational asthma, early removal from exposure and early treatment increase the probability of recovery

> **Most patients with asthma do not need more than low dose ICS**, because at a group level, most of the benefit, including for preventing exacerbations, is obtained at low doses. For ICS doses, see Box 8, p.20.
>
> For most asthma patients, controller treatment can be started with either as-needed low dose ICS-formoterol (or, if not available, low dose ICS whenever SABA is taken) or with regular daily low dose ICS.

Consider starting at a higher step (e.g. medium/high dose ICS, or low-dose ICS-LABA) if on most days the patient has troublesome asthma symptoms; or is waking from asthma once or more a week.

If the initial asthma presentation is with severely uncontrolled asthma, or with an acute exacerbation, give a short course of OCS and start regular controller treatment (e.g. medium dose ICS-LABA).

Consider stepping down after asthma has been well-controlled for 3 months. However, in adults and adolescents, ICS should not be completely stopped.

Before starting initial controller treatment
- Record evidence for the diagnosis of asthma, if possible
- Document symptom control and risk factors
- Assess lung function, when possible
- Train the patient to use the inhaler correctly, and check their technique
- Schedule a follow-up visit.

After starting initial controller treatment
- Review response after 2–3 months, or according to clinical urgency
- See Box 7 for ongoing treatment and other key management issues
- Consider step down when asthma has been well-controlled for 3 months

Box 7. The GINA asthma treatment strategy

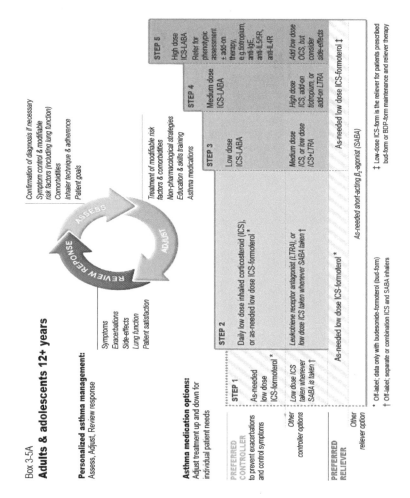

For children 6–11 years, the preferred Step 3 treatment is low dose ICS-LABA or medium dose ICS. For more details about treatment recommendations including in children, supporting evidence, and clinical advice about implementation in different populations see the full GINA 2019 report (www.ginasthma.org). .For more details about Step 5 add-on therapies, see GINA 2019 Pocket Guide on Difficult to Treat and Severe Asthma, and check eligibility criteria with local payers.

Box 8. Low, medium and high daily doses of inhaled corticosteroids

Low dose ICS provides most of the clinical benefit for most patients. However, ICS responsiveness varies between patients, so some patients may need **medium dose ICS** if asthma is uncontrolled despite good adherence and correct inhaler technique with low dose ICS. **High dose ICS** is needed by very few patients, and its long-term use is associated with an increased risk of local and systemic side-effects.

This is not a table of equivalence, but of estimated clinical comparability, based on available studies and product information.

Inhaled corticosteroid	Adults and adolescents		
	Low	Medium	High
Beclometasone dipropionate (CFC)*	200–500	>500–1000	>1000
Beclometasone dipropionate (HFA)	100–200	>200–400	>400
Budesonide (DPI)	200–400	>400–800	>800
Ciclesonide (HFA)	80–160	>160–320	>320
Fluticasone furoate (DPI)	100	n.a.	200
Fluticasone propionate(DPI)	100–250	>250–500	>500
Fluticasone propionate (HFA)	100–250	>250–500	>500
Mometasone furoate	110–220	>220–440	>440
Triamcinolone acetonide	400–1000	>1000–2000	>2000

Inhaled corticosteroid	Children 6-11 years		
	Low	Medium	High
Beclometasone dipropionate (CFC)*	100–200	>200–400	>400
Beclometasone dipropionate (HFA)	50-100	>100-200	>200
Budesonide (DPI)	100–200	>200–400	>400
Budesonide (nebules)	250–500	>500–1000	>1000
Ciclesonide (HFA)	80	>80-160	>160
Fluticasone propionate(DPI)	100–200	>200–400	>400
Fluticasone propionate (HFA)	100–200	>200–500	>500
Mometasone furoate	110	≥220–<440	≥440
Triamcinolone acetonide	400–800	>800–1200	>1200

Doses are in mcg. CFC: chlorofluorocarbon propellant; DPI: dry powder inhaler; HFA: hydrofluoroalkane propellant. *Included for comparison with older literature.

For new preparations, the manufacturer's information should be reviewed carefully, as products containing the same molecule may not be clinically equivalent.

STEPWISE APPROACH FOR ADJUSTING TREATMENT FOR INDIVIDUAL PATIENT NEEDS

Once asthma treatment has been started, ongoing decisions are based on a cycle (Box 6, p.15) to assess the patient, adjust their treatment (pharmacological and non-pharmacological) if needed, and review their response.

The **preferred controller treatments** at each step for adults and adolescents are summarized below and in Box 7 (p.19). For details, including for children 6-11 years, see the full GINA 2019 report. See Box 8 (p.20) for ICS doses.

At each step, **other controller options** are also listed, that are not as effective as the 'preferred controller', but that may be considered for patients with particular risk factors or if the preferred controller is not available.

For patients whose asthma is not well-controlled on a particular treatment, adherence, inhaler technique and comorbidities should be checked before considering a different medication in the same step, or before stepping up.

STEP 1

Preferred controller: As-needed low dose ICS-formoterol (off-label)

Step 1 recommendations are for patients with symptoms less than twice a month and no exacerbation risk factors, a group that is rarely studied.

As-needed low dose ICS-formoterol in Step 1 is supported by *indirect evidence* from a large study of as-needed low-dose budesonide-formoterol compared with SABA-only treatment in patients eligible for Step 2 therapy (O'Byrne et al, NEJMed 2018; see below).

In making this recommendation, the most important considerations were:

- that patients with few interval asthma symptoms can have severe or fatal exacerbations (Dusser et al, Allergy 2007)
- that a 64% reduction in severe exacerbations was found in the Step 2 study with as-needed low dose budesonide-formoterol compared with SABA-only, with <20% of the average ICS dose compared with daily ICS
- the priority to avoid past conflicting messages in which patients were initially told to use SABA for symptom relief, but later had to be told (despite this treatment being effective from their perspective) that they needed to reduce their SABA use by taking a daily controller
- the fact that adherence with ICS is poor in patients with infrequent symptoms, exposing them to risks of SABA-only treatment.

All evidence so far is with low dose budesonide-formoterol, but BDP-formoterol may also be suitable. These medications are well-established for maintenance and reliever therapy in Steps 3-5, and no new safety signals were seen in the as-needed studies with budesonide-formoterol.

Other controller options at Step 1

- *Low dose ICS taken whenever SABA is taken* (off-label): In Step 1, the evidence is again indirect, from studies with separate or combination ICS and SABA inhalers in patients eligible for Step 2 treatment (see below). For this recommendation, the most important considerations were reducing the risk of severe exacerbations, and the difficulty of achieving good adherence with ICS.
- *Daily low dose ICS* had been suggested by GINA since 2014 in Step 1 to reduce the risk of severe exacerbations. However, patients with symptoms less than twice a month are unlikely to take ICS regularly, leaving them exposed to the risks of SABA-only treatment, so it is no longer recommended.

Children 6-11 years

Taking ICS whenever SABA is taken is a possible option, with indirect evidence from a Step 2 study with separate inhalers that showed markedly fewer exacerbations vs SABA-only treatment (Martinez et al, Lancet 2011).

STEP 2

Preferred controllers: Daily low dose ICS plus as-needed SABA, OR as-needed low dose ICS-formoterol *(off-label)*

Daily low dose ICS with as-needed SABA: there is a large body of evidence from RCTs and observational studies showing that the risks of severe exacerbations, hospitalizations and mortality are substantially reduced with regular low dose ICS; symptoms and exercise-induced bronchoconstriction are also reduced. Severe exacerbations are halved even in patients with symptoms 0-1 days a week (Reddel et al, Lancet 2017).

For this recommendation, the most important consideration was reducing the risk of severe exacerbations, but we recognized the problems of poor adherence in mild asthma, exposing patients to SABA-only treatment. The clinician should consider likely adherence before prescribing daily ICS.

As-needed low dose ICS-formoterol *(off-label):* the evidence to date is with low dose budesonide-formoterol. One large study in mild asthma found a 64% reduction in severe exacerbations compared with SABA-only (OByrne et al, NEJMed 2018), and two large studies in mild asthma showed non-inferiority for severe exacerbations compared with regular ICS (O'Byrne et al, NEJMed 2018; Bateman et al, NEJMed 2018).

For this recommendation, the most important considerations were to prevent severe exacerbations and to avoid the need for daily ICS in patients with mild asthma. The small differences in symptom control and lung function compared with daily ICS were considered to be less important, as they were less than the minimal important difference. One study of exercise-induced bronchoconstriction with budesonide-formoterol taken as-needed and before exercise showed similar benefit as daily ICS (Lazarinis et al, Thorax 2014).

Other controller options at Step 2

- *Low dose ICS taken whenever SABA is taken,* either in combination or separate inhalers (off-label). Two studies showed reduced exacerbations compared with SABA-only treatment, one in ages 5-18 years with separate inhalers (Martinez et al, Lancet 2011) and one in adults with combination ICS-SABA (Papi et al, NEJMed 2007). Evidence for similar or fewer exacerbations compared with daily ICS comes from the same studies plus Calhoun et al (JAMA 2012) in adults. In making this recommendation, a high importance was given to preventing severe exacerbations, and a lower importance was given to small differences in symptom control and the inconvenience of needing to carry two inhalers.
- *Leukotriene receptor antagonists (LTRA)* are less effective than regular ICS, particularly for preventing exacerbations.
- *Daily low dose ICS-LABA* as initial therapy leads to faster improvement in symptoms and FEV_1 than ICS alone but is more costly and the exacerbation rate is similar.
- For purely seasonal allergic asthma, evidence is needed. Current advice is to start ICS immediately and cease 4 weeks after end of exposure.

Children 6-11 years

The preferred controller option for children at Step 2 is regular low dose ICS (see Box 8 (p.20) for ICS dose ranges in children). Other less effective controller options for children are daily LTRA, or taking low dose ICS whenever SABA is taken (Martinez et al, Lancet 2011, separate inhalers).

STEP 3

Preferred controller: Low dose ICS-LABA maintenance plus as-needed SABA, OR low dose ICS-formoterol maintenance and reliever therapy

Recommendations in Step 3 are unchanged from 2018. Adherence, inhaler technique and comorbidities should be checked before considering step-up. For patients whose asthma is uncontrolled on low dose ICS, low dose combination ICS-LABA leads to ~20% reduction in exacerbation risk and higher lung function, but little difference in reliever use. For patients with ≥1 exacerbation in the last year, maintenance and reliever treatment with low dose BDP-formoterol or BUD-formoterol is more effective than maintenance ICS-LABA or higher dose ICS with as-needed SABA in reducing severe exacerbations, with a similar level of symptom control.

Other controller options: Medium dose ICS, or low dose ICS plus LTRA. For adult patients with rhinitis who are allergic to house dust mite, consider adding sublingual immunotherapy (SLIT), provided FEV_1 is >70% predicted.

Children (6-11 years): The preferred controller for this age-group is medium dose ICS or low dose ICS-LABA, which have similar benefits.

STEP 4

Preferred controller: Low dose ICS-formoterol maintenance and reliever therapy, OR medium dose ICS-LABA maintenance plus as-needed SABA

Although at a group level most benefit from ICS is obtained at low dose, individual ICS responsiveness varies, and some patients whose asthma is uncontrolled on low dose ICS-LABA despite good adherence and correct technique may benefit from increasing the ICS dose to medium.

Other controller options include: add-on tiotropium by mist inhaler for patients ≥6 years with a history of exacerbations; add-on LTRA; or increasing to high dose ICS-LABA, but with the latter, consider the potential increase in ICS side-effects. For adult patients with rhinitis and asthma who are allergic to house dust mite, consider adding SLIT, provided FEV_1 is >70% predicted.

Children (6-11 years): Continue controller, and refer for expert advice.

STEP 5: Refer for phenotypic investigation ± add-on treatment

Patients with uncontrolled symptoms and/or exacerbations despite Step 4 treatment should be assessed for contributory factors, treatment optimized, and referred for expert assessment including severe asthma phenotype, and potential add-on treatment. The **GINA Pocket Guide on Difficult to Treat and Severe Asthma v2.0 2019** provides a decision tree and practical guide for assessment and management in adults and adolescents. Sputum-guided treatment, if available, improves outcomes in moderate-severe asthma.

Add-on treatments include tiotropium by mist inhaler for patients ≥6 years with a history of exacerbations; for severe allergic asthma, anti-IgE (SC omalizumab, ≥6 years); and for severe eosinophilic asthma, anti-IL5 (SC mepolizumab, ≥6 years, or IV reslizumab, ≥18 years) or anti-IL5R (SC benralizumab, ≥12 years) or anti-IL4R (SC dupilumab, ≥12 years). See glossary (p.33) and check local eligibility criteria for specific add-on therapies.

Other options: Some patients may benefit from low dose OCS but long-term systemic side-effects are common and burdensome.

REVIEWING RESPONSE AND ADJUSTING TREATMENT

How often should patients with asthma be reviewed?

Patients should preferably be seen 1–3 months after starting treatment and every 3–12 months after that, but in pregnancy, asthma should be reviewed every 4–6 weeks. After an exacerbation, a review visit within 1 week should be scheduled. The frequency of review depends on the patient's initial level of symptom control, their risk factors, their response to initial treatment, and their ability and willingness to engage in self-management with an action plan.

Stepping up asthma treatment

Asthma is a variable condition, and periodic adjustment of controller treatment by the clinician and/or patient may be needed.

- *Sustained step-up (for at least 2–3 months)*: if symptoms and/or exacerbations persist despite 2–3 months of controller treatment, assess the following common issues before considering a step-up
  - o Incorrect inhaler technique
  - o Poor adherence
  - o Modifiable risk factors, e.g. smoking
  - o Are symptoms due to comorbid conditions, e.g. allergic rhinitis
- *Short-term step-up (for 1–2 weeks)* by clinician or by patient with written asthma action plan (p29), e.g. during viral infection or allergen exposure
- *Day-to-day adjustment by patient* for patients prescribed as-needed low dose ICS-formoterol for mild asthma, or low dose ICS-formoterol as maintenance and reliever therapy.

Stepping down treatment when asthma is well-controlled

Consider stepping down treatment once good asthma control has been achieved and maintained for 3 months, to find the lowest treatment that controls both symptoms and exacerbations, and minimizes side-effects.

- Choose an appropriate time for step-down (no respiratory infection, patient not travelling, not pregnant)
- Document baseline status (symptom control and lung function), provide a written asthma action plan, monitor closely, and book a follow-up visit
- Step down through available formulations to reduce the ICS dose by 25–50% at 2–3 month intervals (see Box 3-9 in full GINA 2019 report for details of how to step down different controller treatments)
- If asthma is well-controlled on low dose ICS or LTRA, as-needed low dose ICS-formoterol is a step-down option based on two large studies with budesonide-formoterol in adults and adolescents (O'Byrne et al, NEJMed 2018; Bateman et al, NEJMed 2018). Smaller studies have shown that low dose ICS taken whenever SABA is taken (combination or separate inhalers) is more effective as a step-down strategy than SABA alone (Papi et al, NEJMed 2007; Martinez et al, Lancet 2011).
- Do not completely stop ICS in adults or adolescents with a diagnosis of asthma unless this is needed temporarily to confirm the diagnosis of asthma.
- Make sure a follow-up appointment is arranged.

INHALER SKILLS AND ADHERENCE

Provide skills training for effective use of inhaler devices

Most patients (up to 80%) cannot use their inhaler correctly. This contributes to poor symptom control and exacerbations. To ensure effective inhaler use:

- **Choose** the most appropriate device for the patient before prescribing: consider medication, physical problems e.g. arthritis, patient skills, and cost; for ICS by pressurized metered dose inhaler, prescribe a spacer.
- **Check** inhaler technique at every opportunity. Ask the patient to show you how they use the inhaler. Check their technique against a device-specific checklist.
- **Correct** using a physical demonstration, paying attention to incorrect steps. Check technique again, up to 2–3 times if necessary.
- **Confirm** that you have checklists for each of the inhalers you prescribe, and can demonstrate correct technique on them.

Information about inhaler devices and techniques for their use can be found on the GINA website (www.ginasthma.org) and the ADMIT website (www.admit-inhalers.org).

Check and improve adherence with asthma medications

At least 50% of adults and children do not take controller medications as prescribed. Poor adherence contributes to poor symptom control and exacerbations. It may be unintentional (e.g. forgetfulness, cost, misunderstandings) and/or intentional (e.g. not perceiving the need for treatment, fear of side-effects, cultural issues, cost).

To identify patients with adherence problems:

- Ask an empathic question, e.g. "Most patients don't take their inhaler exactly as prescribed. In the last 4 weeks, how many days a week have you been taking it? 0 days a week, or 1, or 2 days [etc]?", or "Do you find it easier to remember your inhaler in the morning or night?"
- Check medication usage, from prescription date, inhaler date/dose counter, dispensing records
- Ask about attitudes and beliefs about asthma and medications

Only a few adherence interventions have been studied closely in asthma and have improved adherence in real-world studies.

- Shared decision-making for medication and dose choice
- Inhaler reminders for missed doses
- Comprehensive asthma education with home visits by asthma nurses
- Clinicians reviewing feedback about their patients' dispensing records
- An automated voice recognition program with telephone messages triggered when refills were due or overdue
- Directly-observed controller therapy at school, with telemedicine oversight

TREATING MODIFIABLE RISK FACTORS

Exacerbation risk can be minimized by optimizing asthma medications, and by identifying and treating modifiable risk factors. Some examples of risk modifiers with consistent high quality evidence are:

- **Guided self-management**: self-monitoring of symptoms and/or PEF, a written asthma action plan (p29), and regular medical review
- **Use of a regimen that minimizes exacerbations**: prescribe an ICS-containing controller, either daily, or, for mild asthma, as-needed ICS-formoterol. For patients with 1 or more exacerbations in the last year, consider a low dose ICS-formoterol maintenance and reliever regimen
- **Avoidance of exposure to tobacco smoke**
- **Confirmed food allergy**: appropriate food avoidance; ensure availability of injectable epinephrine for anaphylaxis
- **For patients with severe asthma**: refer to a specialist center, if available, for detailed assessment and consideration of add-on biologic medications and/or sputum-guided treatment.

NON-PHARMACOLOGICAL STRATEGIES AND INTERVENTIONS

In addition to medications, other therapies and strategies may be considered where relevant, to assist in symptom control and risk reduction. Some examples with consistent high quality evidence are:

- **Smoking cessation advice**: at every visit, strongly encourage smokers to quit. Provide access to counselling and resources. Advise parents and carers to exclude smoking in rooms/cars used by children with asthma
- **Physical activity**: encourage people with asthma to engage in regular physical activity because of its general health benefits. Provide advice about management of exercise-induced bronchoconstriction.
- **Occupational asthma**: ask all patients with adult-onset asthma about their work history. Identify and remove occupational sensitizers as soon as possible. Refer patients for expert advice, if available.
- **NSAIDs including aspirin**: always ask about asthma before prescribing.

Although allergens may contribute to asthma symptoms in sensitized patients, allergen avoidance is not recommended as a general strategy for asthma. These strategies are often complex and expensive, and there are no validated methods for identifying those who are likely to benefit.

Some common triggers for asthma symptoms (e.g. exercise, laughter) should **not** be avoided, and others (e.g. viral respiratory infections, stress) are difficult to avoid and should be managed when they occur.

TREATMENT IN SPECIFIC POPULATIONS OR CONTEXTS

Pregnancy: asthma control often changes during pregnancy. For baby and mother, the advantages of actively treating asthma markedly outweigh any potential risks of usual controller and reliever medications. Down-titration has a low priority in pregnancy. Exacerbations should be treated aggressively.

Rhinitis and sinusitis often coexist with asthma. Chronic rhinosinusitis is associated with more severe asthma. Treatment of allergic rhinitis or chronic rhinosinusitis reduces nasal symptoms but does not improve asthma control.

Obesity: to avoid over- or under-treatment, it is important to document the diagnosis of asthma in the obese. Asthma is more difficult to control in obesity. Weight reduction should be included in the treatment plan for obese patients with asthma; even 5–10% weight loss can improve asthma control.

The elderly: comorbidities and their treatment may complicate asthma management. Factors such as arthritis, eyesight, inspiratory flow, and complexity of treatment regimens should be considered when choosing medications and inhaler devices.

Gastroesophageal reflux (GERD) is commonly seen in asthma. Symptomatic reflux should be treated for its general health benefits, but there is no benefit from treating asymptomatic reflux in asthma.

Anxiety and depression: these are commonly seen in people with asthma, and are associated with worse symptoms and quality of life. Patients should be assisted to distinguish between symptoms of anxiety and of asthma.

Aspirin-exacerbated respiratory disease (AERD): a history of exacerbation following ingestion of aspirin or other NSAIDs is highly suggestive. Patients often have severe asthma and nasal polyposis. Confirmation of the diagnosis of AERD may require challenge in a specialized center with resuscitation facilities, but avoidance of NSAIDs may be recommended on the basis of a clear history. ICS are the mainstay of treatment, but OCS may be required; LTRA may also be useful. Desensitization under specialist care is sometimes effective.

Food allergy and anaphylaxis: food allergy is rarely a trigger for asthma symptoms. It must be assessed with specialist testing. Confirmed food allergy is a risk factor for asthma-related death. Good asthma control is essential; patients should also have an anaphylaxis plan and be trained in appropriate avoidance strategies and use of injectable epinephrine.

Surgery: whenever possible, good asthma control should be achieved pre-operatively. Ensure that controller therapy is maintained throughout the peri-operative period. Patients on long-term high dose ICS, or having more than 2 weeks' OCS in the past 6 months, should receive intra-operative hydrocortisone to reduce the risk of adrenal crisis.

ASTHMA FLARE-UPS (EXACERBATIONS)

A flare-up or exacerbation is an acute or sub-acute worsening in symptoms and lung function from the patient's usual status; occasionally it may be the initial presentation of asthma.

For discussion with patients, the word 'flare-up' is preferred. 'Episodes', 'attacks' and 'acute severe asthma' are often used, but they have variable meanings, particularly for patients.

The management of worsening asthma and exacerbations should be considered as a continuum, from self-management by the patient with a written asthma action plan, through to management of more severe symptoms in primary care, the emergency department and in hospital.

Identifying patients at risk of asthma-related death

Patients with features indicating increased risk of asthma-related death should be flagged for more frequent review. These features include:

- *History*: A history of near-fatal asthma (ever) requiring intubation and ventilation; hospitalization or emergency care for asthma in the last year
- *Medications*: not currently using ICS, or with poor adherence with ICS; currently using or recently stopped OCS (an indication of recent severity); over-use of SABA, especially more than 1 canister per month
- *Comorbidities*: history of psychiatric disease or psychosocial problems; confirmed food allergy in a patient with asthma
- Lack of a written asthma action plan

WRITTEN ASTHMA ACTION PLANS

All patients should be provided with a written asthma action plan appropriate for their level of asthma control and health literacy, so they know how to recognize and respond to worsening asthma.

Box 9. Self-management with a written action plan

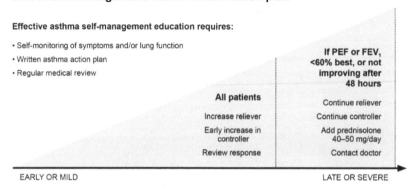

Effective asthma self-management education requires:

- Self-monitoring of symptoms and/or lung function
- Written asthma action plan
- Regular medical review

If PEF or FEV,
<60% best, or not
improving after
48 hours

All patients

Increase reliever

Early increase in controller

Review response

Continue reliever

Continue controller

Add prednisolone
40–50 mg/day

Contact doctor

EARLY OR MILD   LATE OR SEVERE

The written asthma action plan should include:

- The patient's usual asthma medications
- When and how to increase medications, and start OCS
- How to access medical care if symptoms fail to respond

Action plans can be based on symptoms and/or (in adults) PEF. Patients who deteriorate quickly should be advised to seek urgent care immediately.

Medication changes for written asthma action plans (see GINA Box 4-2)

Increase frequency of inhaled reliever (SABA, or low dose ICS-formoterol); add spacer for pMDI.

Increase controller: Rapid increase in controller, depending on usual controller medication and regimen, as follows:

- *ICS*: In adults and adolescents, quadruple dose. However, in children with good adherence, 5x increase is not effective..
- *Maintenance ICS-formoterol*: Quadruple maintenance ICS-formoterol dose (to maximum formoterol dose of 72 mcg/day).
- *Maintenance ICS-other LABA*: Step up to higher dose formulation, or consider adding separate ICS inhaler to achieve quadruple ICS dose.
- *Maintenance and reliever ICS-formoterol*: Continue maintenance dose; increase reliever doses as needed (maximum formoterol 72 mcg/day).

Oral corticosteroids (preferably morning dosing; review before ceasing):

- Adults - prednisolone 40-50mg, usually for 5–7 days.
- For children, 1–2 mg/kg/day up to 40mg, usually for 3–5 days.
- Tapering not needed if OCS has been given for less than 2 weeks.

MANAGING EXACERBATIONS IN PRIMARY OR ACUTE CARE

Assess exacerbation severity while starting SABA and oxygen. Assess dyspnea (e.g. is the patient able to speak sentences, or only words), respiratory rate, pulse rate, oxygen saturation and lung function (e.g. PEF). Check for anaphylaxis.

Consider alternative causes of acute breathlessness (e.g. heart failure, upper airway dysfunction, inhaled foreign body or pulmonary embolism).

Arrange immediate transfer to an acute care facility if there are signs of severe exacerbation, or to intensive care if the patient is drowsy, confused, or has a silent chest. For these patients, immediately give inhaled SABA, inhaled ipratropium bromide, oxygen and systemic corticosteroids.

Start treatment with repeated doses of SABA (usually by pMDI and spacer), early OCS, and controlled flow oxygen if available. Check response of symptoms and saturation frequently, and measure lung function after 1 hour. Titrate oxygen to maintain saturation of 93–95% in adults and adolescents (94–98% in children 6–12 years).

Box 10. Management of asthma exacerbations in primary care

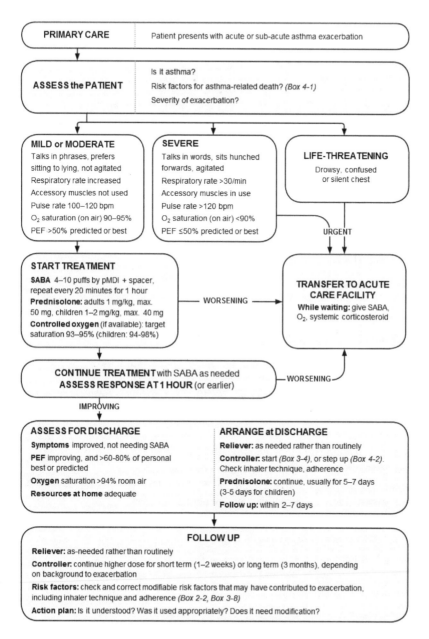

O$_2$: oxygen; PEF: peak expiratory flow; SABA: short-acting beta$_2$-agonist (doses are for salbutamol)

For severe exacerbations, add ipratropium bromide, and consider giving SABA by nebulizer. In acute care facilities, intravenous magnesium sulfate may be considered for inadequate response to intensive initial treatment.

Do not routinely perform chest X-ray or blood gases, or routinely prescribe antibiotics, for asthma exacerbations.

REVIEWING RESPONSE

Monitor patients closely and frequently during treatment, and titrate treatment according to response. Transfer to higher level care if worsening or failing to respond. Decide on need for hospitalization based on clinical status, symptoms and lung function, response to treatment, recent and past history of exacerbations, and ability to manage at home.

Before discharge, arrange ongoing treatment. For most patients, prescribe regular controller therapy (or increase current dose) to reduce the risk of further exacerbations. Continue increased controller doses for 2–4 weeks, and reduce reliever to as-needed dosing. Check inhaler technique and adherence. Provide an interim written asthma action plan.

Arrange early follow-up after any exacerbation, within 2–7 days (for children, within 1-2 working days). Consider early referral for specialist advice after hospitalization, or for patients with repeated ED presentations.

FOLLOW-UP AFTER AN EXACERBATION

Exacerbations often represent failures in chronic asthma care, and they provide opportunities to review the patient's asthma management. All patients must be followed up regularly by a health care provider until symptoms and lung function return to normal.

Take the opportunity to review:
- The patient's understanding of the cause of the exacerbation
- Modifiable risk factors for exacerbations, e.g. smoking
- Understanding of purposes of medications, and inhaler technique skills. Adherence with ICS and OCS may fall rapidly after discharge.
- Review and revise written asthma action plan

Comprehensive post-discharge programs that include optimal controller management, inhaler technique, self-monitoring, written asthma action plan and regular review are cost-effective and are associated with significant improvement in asthma outcomes.

Referral for expert advice should be considered for patients who have been hospitalized for asthma, or who re-present for acute asthma care. Patients who have had >1-2 exacerbations/year despite Step 4-5 treatment should be referred (see GINA Pocket Guide on Difficult to Treat and Severe Asthma).

GLOSSARY OF ASTHMA MEDICATION CLASSES

For more details, see full GINA 2019 report and Appendix (www.ginasthma.org) and Product Information from manufacturers. *Check local eligibility criteria from payers.

Medications	Action and use	Adverse effects
CONTROLLER MEDICATIONS		
Inhaled corticosteroids (ICS)		
(pMDIs or DPIs) e.g. beclometasone, budesonide, ciclesonide, fluticasone propionate, fluticasone furoate, mometasone, triamcinolone	ICS are the most effective anti-inflammatory medications for asthma. ICS reduce symptoms, increase lung function, improve quality of life, and reduce the risk of exacerbations and asthma-related hospitalizations and death. ICS differ in their potency and bioavailability, but most of the benefit is seen at low doses (see Box 8 (p.20) for low, medium and high doses of different ICS).	Most patients using ICS do not experience side-effects. Local side-effects include oropharyngeal candidiasis and dysphonia; these can be reduced by use of a spacer with pMDIs, and rinsing with water and spitting out after inhalation. Long-term high doses increase the risk of systemic side-effects such as osteoporosis, cataract and glaucoma.
ICS and long-acting beta$_2$ agonist bronchodilator combinations (ICS-LABA)		
(pMDIs or DPIs) e.g. beclometasone-formoterol, budesonide-formoterol, fluticasone furoate-vilanterol, fluticasone propionate formoterol, fluticasone propionate-salmeterol, and mometasone-formoterol.	When a low dose of ICS alone fails to achieve good control of asthma, the addition of LABA to ICS improves symptoms, lung function and reduces exacerbations in more patients, more rapidly, than doubling the dose of ICS. Two regimens are available: low-dose combination beclometasone or budesonide with low dose formoterol for maintenance and reliever treatment, and maintenance ICS-LABA with SABA as reliever. Maintenance and reliever treatment with low dose ICS-formoterol reduces exacerbations compared with conventional maintenance therapy with SABA as reliever.	The LABA component may be associated with tachycardia, headache or cramps. Current recommendations are that LABA and ICS are safe for asthma when used in combination. LABA should not be used without ICS in asthma due to increased risk of serious adverse outcomes.
Leukotriene modifiers		
(tablets) e.g. montelukast, pranlukast, zafirlukast, zileuton	Target one part of the inflammatory pathway in asthma. Used as an option for controller therapy, particularly in children. Used alone: less effective than low dose ICS; added to ICS: less effective than ICS-LABA.	Few side-effects in placebo-controlled studies except elevated liver function tests with zileuton and zafirlukast.
Chromones		
(pMDIs or DPIs) e.g. sodium cromoglycate and nedocromil sodium	Very limited role in long-term treatment of asthma. Weak anti-inflammatory effect, less effective than low-dose ICS. Require meticulous inhaler maintenance.	Side effects are uncommon but include cough upon inhalation and pharyngeal discomfort.

Medications	Action and use	Adverse effects
ADD-ON CONTROLLER MEDICATIONS		
Long-acting anticholinergic		
(tiotropium, mist inhaler, ≥6 years*)	An add-on option at Step 4 or 5 by mist inhaler for patients with a history of exacerbations despite ICS ± LABA*	Side-effects are uncommon but include dry mouth.
Anti-IgE		
(omalizumab, SC, ≥6 years*)	An add-on option for patients with severe allergic asthma uncontrolled on high dose ICS-LABA*. Self-administration may be permitted*	Reactions at the site of injection are common but minor. Anaphylaxis is rare.
Anti-IL5 and anti-IL5R		
(anti-IL5 mepolizumab [SC, ≥12 years*] or reslizumab [IV, ≥18 years], or anti-IL5 receptor benralizumab [SC, ≥12 years]	Add-on options for patients with severe eosinophilic asthma uncontrolled on high dose ICS-LABA*	Headache, and reactions at injection site are common but minor.
Anti-IL4R		
(dupilumab, SC, ≥12 years*)	An add-on option for patients with severe eosinophilic or Type 2 asthma uncontrolled on high dose ICS-LABA, or requiring maintenance OCS. Also approved for treatment of moderate-severe atopic dermatitis. Self-administration may be permitted*	Reactions at injection site are common but minor. Blood eosinophilia occurs in 4-13% of patients
Systemic corticosteroids		
(tablets,suspension or intramuscular (IM) or intravenous (IV) injection) e.g. prednisone, prednisolone, methylprednisolone, hydrocortisone	Short-term treatment (usually 5–7 days in adults) is important in the treatment of severe acute exacerbations, with main effects seen after 4–6 hours. Oral corticosteroid (OCS) therapy is preferred to IM or IV therapy and is effective in preventing relapse. Tapering is required if treatment given for more than 2 weeks. Long-term treatment with OCS may be required for some patients with severe asthma, but side-effects must be taken into account.	Short-term use: some adverse effects e.g. sleep disturbance, reflux, appetite increase, hyperglycaemia, mood changes. Long-term use: limited by significant systemic adverse effects e.g. cataract, glaucoma, hypertension, diabetes, adrenal suppression osteoporosis. Assess for osteoporosis risk and treat appropriately.

Medications	Action and use	Adverse effects
RELIEVER MEDICATIONS		
Short-acting inhaled beta$_2$-agonist bronchodilators (SABA)		
(pMDIs, DPIs and, rarely, solution for nebulization or injection) e.g. salbutamol (albuterol), terbutaline.	Inhaled SABAs provide quick relief of asthma symptoms and bronchoconstriction including in acute exacerbations, and for pre-treatment of exercise-induced bronchoconstriction. SABAs should be used only as-needed and at the lowest dose and frequency required.	Tremor and tachycardia are commonly reported with initial use of SABA. Tolerance develops rapidly with regular use. Excess use, or poor response indicate poor asthma control.
Low-dose ICS-formoterol		
(beclometasone-formoterol or budesonide-formoterol)	Low dose budesonide-formoterol or BDP formoterol is the reliever for patients prescribed as-needed controller therapy for mild asthma, where it substantially reduces the risk of severe exacerbations compared with SABA-only treatment. It is also used as the reliever for patients with moderate-severe asthma prescribed maintenance and reliever treatment, where it reduces the risk of exacerbations compared with using as-needed SABA, with similar symptom control.	As for ICS-LABA above
Short-acting anticholinergics		
(pMDIs or DPIs) e.g. ipratropium bromide, oxitropium bromide	Long-term use: ipratropium is a less effective reliever medication than SABAs. Short-term use in acute asthma: inhaled ipratropium added to SABA reduces the risk of hospital admission	Dryness of the mouth or a bitter taste.

ACKNOWLEDGEMENTS

The activities of the Global Initiative of Asthma are supported by the work of members of the GINA Board of Directors and Committees (listed below), and by the sale of GINA products. The members of the GINA committees are solely responsible for the statements and recommendations presented in this and other GINA publications.

GINA Science Committee (2019)

Helen Reddel*, Australia, *Chair*; Leonard Bacharier, USA; Eric Bateman, South Africa.; Allan Becker, Canada; Louis-Philippe Boulet*, Canada; Guy Brusselle, Belgium; Roland Buhl, Germany; Louise Fleming, UK; Johan de Jongste, The Netherlands; J. Mark FitzGerald, Canada; Hiromasa Inoue, Japan; Fanny Wai-san Ko, Hong Kong; Jerry Krishnan*, USA; Søren Pedersen, Denmark; Aziz Sheikh, UK.

GINA Board of Directors (2019)

Louis-Philippe Boulet*, Canada, *Chair;* Eric Bateman, South Africa; Guy Brusselle, Belgium; Alvaro Cruz*, Brazil; J Mark FitzGerald, Canada; Hiromasa Inoue, Japan; Jerry Krishnan*, USA; Mark Levy*, United Kingdom; Jiangtao Lin, China; Søren Pedersen, Denmark; Helen Reddel*, Australia; Arzu Yorgancioglu*, Turkey.

GINA Dissemination and Implementation Committee (2019)

Mark Levy, UK, *Chair;* other members indicated by asterisks (*) above.

GINA Assembly

The GINA Assembly includes members from 45 countries. Their names are listed on the GINA website, www.ginasthma.org.

GINA Program Director: Rebecca Decker, USA

GINA PUBLICATIONS

- **Global Strategy for Asthma Management and Prevention** (updated 2019). This report provides an integrated approach to asthma that can be adapted for a wide range of health systems. The report has a user-friendly format with many practical summary tables and flow-charts for use in clinical practice. It is updated yearly.
- **GINA Online Appendix** (updated 2019). Detailed information to support the main GINA report. Updated yearly.
- **Pocket Guide for asthma management and prevention for adults and children older than 5 years** (updated 2019). Summary for primary health care providers, to be used in conjunction with the main GINA report.
- **Pocket guide for asthma management and prevention in children 5 years and younger** (to be updated 2019). A summary of patient care information about pre-schoolers with asthma or wheeze, to be used in conjunction with the main GINA 2019 report.
- **Diagnosis of asthma-COPD overlap** (updated 2018). This is a stand-alone copy of the corresponding chapter in the main GINA report. It is co-published by GINA and GOLD (the Global Initiative for Chronic Obstructive Lung Disease, www.goldcopd.org).
- **A toolbox of clinical practice aids and implementation tools** is available on the GINA website.

GINA publications and other resources are available from www.ginasthma.org

CPSIA information can be obtained
at www.ICGtesting.com
Printed in the USA
LVHW071937030520
654938LV00004B/385